OPTIMIZING PULMONARY HYPERTENSION

A Comprehensive Guide to Dietary Strategies for Better Health

Dr. Raymond F. Bernard

Disclaimer: the opinion and views expressed in this book are those of the author and do not necessarily reflect the policy or position of any character or organization mention in this book

TABLE OF CONTENTS

CHAPTER 1

Introduction to Pulmonary Hypertension and Diet

In this chapter, we delve into the complex and often misunderstood world of pulmonary hypertension (PH) and its close relationship with diet. We'll explore how PH affects the body, why nutrition plays a pivotal role in managing this condition, and the overall importance of making informed dietary choices for individuals living with PH.

Understanding Pulmonary Hypertension (PH)

Pulmonary hypertension is a medical condition characterized by high blood pressure in the pulmonary arteries, the vessels that carry oxygen-poor blood from the heart to the lungs for oxygenation. Unlike systemic hypertension, which affects the entire body's circulation, pulmonary hypertension specifically targets the pulmonary circulation, making it a distinct and challenging condition.

PH occurs when the pulmonary arteries narrow, thicken, or

become blocked, which forces the right side of the heart to work harder to pump blood through these vessels. Over time, this increased workload can lead to heart strain and potentially heart failure.

There are several types of pulmonary hypertension, each with its unique underlying causes. These may include idiopathic pulmonary arterial hypertension (IPAH), which has no known cause, or secondary PH, which is a result of other medical conditions like heart or lung diseases. Regardless of the type, PH shares common symptoms such as shortness of breath, fatigue, chest pain, and swelling in the ankles and legs.

The Role of Diet in Managing PH

Now, let's explore why diet is of such importance in managing pulmonary hypertension. To appreciate this, we must understand the following key factors:

1. **Fluid and Sodium Balance**: PH patients often face issues with fluid retention. This means that

the body can accumulate excess fluid, causing swelling and worsening of symptoms. Sodium (salt) intake directly affects fluid retention. Therefore, managing sodium intake is critical for PH patients to maintain a balanced fluid level.

2. **Nutrient Density**: Since PH can result in decreased oxygen levels in the blood, it's crucial to consume foods rich in nutrients, especially those that aid in oxygen transport, energy production, and overall cardiovascular health. These

nutrients include iron, B vitamins, and antioxidants.

3. **Heart Health**: PH places extra strain on the right side of the heart. A heart-healthy diet is essential to support this vital organ. Such a diet emphasizes lean proteins, healthy fats, whole grains, and plenty of fruits and vegetables.

4. **Medication Interactions**: Some medications commonly prescribed for PH may have specific dietary restrictions or interactions. Understanding how these drugs work in conjunction

with your diet is crucial for their effectiveness and safety.

5. **Weight Management**: Maintaining a healthy weight is essential for PH patients. Excess weight can worsen PH symptoms and strain the heart. A balanced diet helps manage weight and support overall health.

6. **Energy Levels**: PH can be physically taxing, leading to fatigue and reduced energy levels. Proper nutrition can help boost energy and alleviate these symptoms.

Importance of Making Informed Dietary Choices

The link between PH and diet underscores the importance of making informed dietary choices. For PH patients, what they eat directly impacts their quality of life. Let's delve into a few key aspects:

Sodium Intake: Sodium is a critical factor for PH patients due to its impact on fluid retention. Excess sodium can lead to swelling and increased strain on the heart. Therefore, it's essential to reduce sodium intake by avoiding highly processed, salty foods and focusing on fresh, whole ingredients.

Fluid Management: Monitoring fluid intake is equally important. While staying hydrated is crucial, excessive fluid consumption can lead to discomfort and worsen symptoms. Balancing fluid intake with the advice of a healthcare provider is vital.

Balanced Nutrition: A balanced diet provides the body with essential nutrients needed for overall health. This includes lean proteins, healthy fats, complex carbohydrates, and a variety of vitamins and minerals. Lean proteins, such as poultry, fish, and legumes, help maintain muscle strength, while healthy fats, like those found in avocados and nuts, support heart health.

Mindful Eating: Mindful eating is a practice that involves paying close attention to the act of eating, savoring each bite, and recognizing hunger and fullness cues. For PH patients, mindful eating can help prevent overeating, support digestion, and enhance the overall dining experience.

Medication Management: Some medications used to treat

PH can interact with certain foods or nutrients. Patients should work closely with their healthcare team to understand these interactions and adjust their diets accordingly.

Supporting Heart Health: The strain placed on the heart by PH requires special attention to cardiovascular health. This can be achieved by reducing saturated and trans fats, incorporating heart-healthy foods like oats and berries, and maintaining an appropriate calorie intake.

In conclusion, Chapter 1 lays the foundation for understanding the profound impact of diet on pulmonary hypertension. By comprehending the relationship between PH and nutrition, patients can embark on a journey toward better symptom management and an improved quality of life. It underscores the importance of making informed dietary choices that align with the specific needs of individuals living with PH. Throughout the subsequent chapters of this cookbook, we will explore practical ways to put this knowledge into action, providing delicious and nutritious recipes tailored to the unique requirements of PH patients.

CHAPTER 2

Building a PH-Friendly Kitchen

In this chapter, we venture into the heart of your culinary journey in managing pulmonary hypertension (PH) by exploring how to set up a PH-friendly kitchen. This isn't just about the physical layout of your kitchen but also about stocking it with the right ingredients, tools, and resources to ensure that cooking for your specific needs becomes not only manageable but also enjoyable.

The PH-Friendly Kitchen: An Introduction

Imagine your kitchen as the canvas upon which you'll paint the masterpiece of your PH-friendly diet. Just as a painter needs the right brushes, colors, and inspiration, you need the right tools and ingredients to craft nourishing and satisfying meals that support your health.

Stocking Your Pantry with PH-Friendly Ingredients

1. **Low-Sodium Staples**: Sodium is a key player in fluid retention, which can exacerbate PH symptoms. Stock up on low-sodium alternatives like low-sodium broths, canned vegetables without added salt, and herbs and spices for flavor.

2. **Whole Grains**: Whole grains like brown rice, quinoa, and whole wheat pasta provide a good source of fiber and energy, helping you feel fuller for longer and maintaining stable blood sugar levels.

3. **Lean Proteins**: Choose lean protein sources like skinless poultry, fish, tofu, and legumes. These are essential for muscle strength and repair.

4. **Healthy Fats**: Incorporate sources of healthy fats such as olive oil, avocados, and nuts. These fats support heart health and can add richness and flavor to your dishes.

5. **Fresh Fruits and Vegetables**: Opt for a variety of fresh produce, including leafy greens, colorful bell peppers, and

antioxidant-rich berries. These provide essential vitamins and minerals while adding vibrant color and flavor to your meals.

6. **Low-Sugar Options**: Be mindful of added sugars in packaged foods. Look for low-sugar or no-sugar-added versions of products like cereals and sauces.

7. **PH-Friendly Snacks**: Keep healthy snacks on hand for when hunger strikes between meals. This can include unsalted nuts, yogurt, or fresh fruit.

Essential Kitchen Tools for PH Patients

Now that you've stocked your pantry, it's time to ensure your kitchen is equipped with the necessary tools to make cooking for PH management a breeze:

1. **Food Scale**: Precision in measuring ingredients is crucial, especially when it comes to sodium intake and portion control.

2. **Measuring Cups and Spoons**: These are essential for accurately measuring ingredients for recipes.

3. **Quality Knives**: Invest in good-quality knives to make chopping and slicing easier and safer.

4. **Non-Stick Cookware**: Non-stick pots and pans require less oil for cooking and are easier to clean, making them a valuable addition to your kitchen.

5. **Blender or Food Processor**: These are versatile tools for creating smoothies, soups, and sauces with a smooth texture.

6. **Steamer**: Steaming vegetables is a great way to

retain their nutrients while minimizing the need for added fats.

7. **Herbs and Spices**: Build a collection of herbs and spices to add flavor to your dishes without relying on salt. Some excellent options include basil, oregano, thyme, and garlic powder.

Tips for Meal Planning and Organization

Efficient meal planning can simplify your culinary journey while ensuring that you consistently follow a PH-friendly diet. Here are some tips:

1. **Weekly Meal Plans**: Plan your meals for the week ahead. This helps you create balanced, PH-friendly menus and minimizes last-minute, less healthy choices.

2. **Batch Cooking**: Cook larger quantities of PH-friendly dishes and freeze individual portions. This way, you'll have convenient, homemade meals at your fingertips when you're short on time or energy.

3. **Labeling**: Label containers with the date and contents to avoid confusion and prevent food waste.

4. **Inventory Check**: Regularly assess your pantry and refrigerator to avoid overbuying or running out of essential ingredients.

5. **Cooking Schedule**: Establish a cooking routine that works for your schedule. Some people prefer to cook several meals on one day, while others prefer daily cooking.

6. **Experiment with Recipes**: Don't be afraid to experiment with new recipes and ingredients. Variety is key to a satisfying PH-friendly diet.

By setting up a PH-friendly kitchen, you're not only preparing yourself for success in managing your condition but also creating an environment where you can truly enjoy the process of cooking. This chapter lays the groundwork for the culinary adventures that lie ahead in this cookbook, ensuring that your kitchen becomes a sanctuary for creating delicious and nutritious meals that support your health and well-being.

CHAPTER 3

PH-Friendly Breakfasts

In Chapter 3, we venture into the realm of breakfast, often considered the most important meal of the day. For individuals managing pulmonary hypertension (PH), a balanced and energizing breakfast is crucial to start the day on the right foot. We will explore why breakfast is essential, delve into the nutritional requirements, and provide a variety of PH-friendly breakfast options that are both delicious and nourishing.

The Significance of Breakfast for PH Patients

Breakfast plays a pivotal role in supporting individuals with pulmonary hypertension. Here's why:

1. **Energy Boost**: Breakfast jumpstarts your metabolism and provides the necessary energy to fuel your body for the day ahead. For PH patients who often contend with fatigue, this boost is especially valuable.

2. **Blood Sugar Regulation**: Eating a balanced breakfast helps maintain stable blood sugar levels, preventing energy crashes and mood swings.

3. **Medication Compatibility**: Many medications prescribed for PH are taken in the morning. Having breakfast ensures you're well-fueled for any potential side effects and aids in medication absorption.

4. **Nutrient Intake**: A nutritious breakfast provides essential vitamins and

minerals, supporting overall health and helping manage specific dietary requirements related to PH.

Nutritional Considerations for PH-Friendly Breakfasts

Before we dive into delicious breakfast ideas, let's explore the nutritional requirements for individuals with pulmonary hypertension:

1. **Protein**: Including a source of lean protein in your breakfast is essential for muscle maintenance and overall strength. Options like

Greek yogurt, eggs, tofu, or lean turkey sausages are great choices.

2. **Complex Carbohydrates**: Whole grains like oats, whole wheat bread, or quinoa provide sustained energy throughout the morning and are rich in fiber, aiding in digestion.

3. **Healthy Fats**: Incorporating sources of healthy fats such as avocados, nuts, or chia seeds can add richness and flavor to your breakfast while supporting heart health.

4. **Fruits and Vegetables**: Fresh or frozen fruits and vegetables provide essential vitamins, minerals, and antioxidants. They also add natural sweetness and vibrancy to your morning meal.

5. **Low-Sodium Options**: PH patients should be mindful of sodium intake. Opt for low-sodium versions of ingredients like bread, canned vegetables, and seasonings.

Now, let's explore some PH-friendly breakfast options:

1. Oatmeal with Fresh Berries and Almonds

Ingredients:

- 1/2 cup rolled oats
- 1 cup unsweetened almond milk
- 1/2 cup fresh berries (e.g., strawberries, blueberries)
- 1 tablespoon chopped almonds
- 1 teaspoon honey (optional)

Instructions:

- Cook the oats in almond milk until they reach your desired consistency.

- Top with fresh berries, chopped almonds, and a drizzle of honey if desired.

2. Scrambled Tofu with Spinach and Tomatoes

Ingredients:

- 1/2 cup crumbled firm tofu
- 1 cup fresh spinach
- 1/2 cup diced tomatoes
- 1/4 teaspoon turmeric (for color)
- Salt and pepper to taste
- 1 teaspoon olive oil

Instructions:

- Heat olive oil in a pan and add crumbled tofu.
- Add turmeric, salt, and pepper for flavor.
- Cook until tofu begins to brown.
- Add spinach and tomatoes, cooking until spinach wilts.

3. Greek Yogurt Parfait with Mixed Fruit

Ingredients:

- 1/2 cup Greek yogurt (low-fat or non-fat)
- 1/2 cup mixed fruit (e.g., kiwi, banana, pineapple)

- 1 tablespoon chopped walnuts
- 1 teaspoon honey (optional)

Instructions:

- Layer Greek yogurt, mixed fruit, and chopped walnuts in a glass.
- Drizzle with honey for extra sweetness if desired.

4. Peanut Butter Banana Smoothie

Ingredients:

- 1 ripe banana
- 2 tablespoons peanut butter (unsalted)

- 1 cup unsweetened almond milk
- 1/2 cup rolled oats
- 1/2 teaspoon cinnamon
- Ice cubes (optional)

Instructions:

- Blend banana, peanut butter, almond milk, oats, and cinnamon until smooth.
- Add ice cubes if you prefer a colder texture.

5. Veggie Breakfast Burrito

Ingredients:

- 2 scrambled eggs (or tofu scramble)

- 1 whole wheat tortilla
- 1/4 cup diced bell peppers
- 1/4 cup diced tomatoes
- 2 tablespoons chopped spinach
- Salsa (low-sodium) for dipping

Instructions:

- Lay out the tortilla and place scrambled eggs (or tofu) in the center.
- Add diced vegetables on top.
- Roll up the tortilla, folding in the sides as you go.
- Serve with salsa for dipping.

These breakfast options are not only delicious but also tailored to meet the nutritional needs of PH patients. They provide the necessary nutrients, including protein, complex carbohydrates, healthy fats, vitamins, and minerals, to support your overall health and well-being.

In conclusion, Chapter 3 sets the stage for your daily culinary journey by emphasizing the importance of a nourishing breakfast for pulmonary hypertension patients. With these PH-friendly breakfast ideas, you'll have the tools to start your day with energy, positivity, and a commitment to managing your condition through a well-balanced diet. Remember to consult with your healthcare team for personalized dietary guidance and adjustments based on your specific needs.

CHAPTER 4

PH-Safe Lunches

In Chapter 4, we turn our attention to lunch, a meal that can often be challenging for individuals managing pulmonary hypertension (PH). We will explore the significance of well-balanced lunches in the context of PH management, delve into the nutritional considerations, and provide a variety of PH-safe lunch ideas that are both nourishing and satisfying.

The Role of Lunch in PH Management

Lunch is a crucial part of your daily nutrition, and for PH patients, it serves multiple purposes:

1. **Energy Replenishment**: Lunch provides a midday energy boost, combating fatigue and ensuring you remain active throughout the day.

2. **Blood Sugar Control**: Eating a balanced lunch helps maintain stable blood sugar levels, preventing

energy crashes and mood swings.

3. **Medication Timing**: Many medications prescribed for PH may need to be taken with food. Having a substantial lunch ensures that your medications are effectively absorbed.

4. **Nutrient Intake**: A nutritious lunch contributes to your overall daily intake of essential nutrients. For those with PH, this supports the specific dietary requirements of managing the condition.

Nutritional Considerations for PH-Safe Lunches

Before we dive into some lunch ideas, let's explore the key nutritional elements that should be included in a PH-safe lunch:

1. **Lean Protein**: Incorporate a source of lean protein in your lunch to support muscle maintenance and repair. Options include skinless poultry, fish, lean beef, tofu, or legumes.

2. **Complex Carbohydrates**: Whole grains such as brown rice, quinoa, or whole wheat bread provide sustained

energy and are rich in fiber, aiding in digestion.

3. **Healthy Fats**: Include sources of healthy fats like avocados, nuts, or olive oil to support heart health and add flavor and richness to your meal.

4. **Fruits and Vegetables**: Fresh or cooked vegetables and fruits are rich in vitamins, minerals, and antioxidants, adding color and vibrancy to your lunch while supporting overall health.

5. **Low-Sodium Options**: PH patients should be mindful

of sodium intake to manage fluid retention. Opt for low-sodium ingredients and seasonings.

Now, let's explore some PH-safe lunch ideas:

1. Grilled Chicken and Vegetable Wrap

Ingredients:

- 4 oz grilled chicken breast (sliced)
- Whole wheat tortilla
- 1/2 cup mixed grilled vegetables (bell peppers, zucchini, onions)

- 2 tablespoons hummus (low-sodium)
- Fresh spinach leaves

Instructions:

- Lay out the whole wheat tortilla.
- Spread a layer of hummus on the tortilla.
- Add sliced grilled chicken, mixed grilled vegetables, and fresh spinach.
- Roll up the tortilla and cut in half for a satisfying wrap.

2. Quinoa and Black Bean Salad

Ingredients:

- 1 cup cooked quinoa
- 1/2 cup canned black beans (rinsed and drained)
- 1/2 cup diced tomatoes
- 1/4 cup diced red onion
- 1/4 cup chopped fresh cilantro
- Juice of 1 lime
- 1 tablespoon olive oil
- Salt and pepper to taste

Instructions:

- In a large bowl, combine cooked quinoa, black beans, diced tomatoes, red onion, and cilantro.
- In a small bowl, whisk together lime juice, olive oil,

salt, and pepper to create the dressing.

- Pour the dressing over the salad and toss to combine.

3. Spinach and Strawberry Salad with Grilled Salmon

Ingredients:

- 4 oz grilled salmon fillet
- 2 cups fresh spinach leaves
- 1/2 cup sliced strawberries
- 2 tablespoons chopped almonds
- Balsamic vinaigrette dressing (low-sodium)

Instructions:

- In a large bowl, combine fresh spinach, sliced strawberries, and chopped almonds.
- Drizzle with balsamic vinaigrette dressing and toss to coat.
- Top with grilled salmon for a protein-rich salad.

4. Lentil and Vegetable Soup

Ingredients:

- 1 cup cooked lentils
- 1/2 cup diced carrots
- 1/2 cup diced celery
- 1/2 cup diced onions
- 2 cloves garlic (minced)

- 4 cups low-sodium vegetable broth
- 1 teaspoon olive oil
- 1 bay leaf
- Salt and pepper to taste

Instructions:

- In a large pot, heat olive oil and sauté diced onions, carrots, and celery until softened.
- Add minced garlic and cook for an additional minute.
- Add cooked lentils, vegetable broth, bay leaf, salt, and pepper.
- Simmer for 15-20 minutes until vegetables are tender.

5. Turkey and Avocado Lettuce Wraps

Ingredients:

- Romaine lettuce leaves
- 4 oz sliced turkey breast
- 1/2 avocado (sliced)
- 1/4 cup diced tomatoes
- 2 tablespoons Greek yogurt (low-fat)

Instructions:

- Lay out romaine lettuce leaves as wraps.
- Add sliced turkey, avocado, diced tomatoes, and a dollop of Greek yogurt to each leaf.

- Roll up the lettuce wraps and secure with toothpicks if needed.

These lunch ideas offer a balance of protein, complex carbohydrates, healthy fats, and plenty of vegetables and fruits while keeping sodium in check. They provide you with a satisfying and nourishing midday meal, which is essential for managing your PH and maintaining your overall health and well-being.

In conclusion, Chapter 4 highlights the importance of well-balanced lunches in the context of pulmonary hypertension management. By focusing on these PH-safe lunch ideas, you can ensure that your midday meal not only supports your specific dietary needs but also adds variety and enjoyment to your daily diet. As always, consult with your healthcare team for personalized dietary guidance tailored to your individual requirements and preferences.

CHAPTER 5

Heart-Healthy Dinners

In Chapter 5, we delve into the world of dinner, a meal often associated with family gatherings and relaxation after a long day. For individuals managing pulmonary hypertension (PH), crafting heart-healthy dinners is essential for managing symptoms and supporting overall well-being. This chapter explores why dinner is crucial, delves into key nutritional considerations, and provides a range of delicious PH-friendly dinner ideas.

The Importance of Heart-Healthy Dinners for PH Patients

Dinner holds a special place in your daily nutrition, especially for those with pulmonary hypertension, for several reasons:

1. **Evening Energy**: Dinner provides the energy needed to stay active and alert during the evening hours, ensuring you can enjoy your evening without feeling fatigued.

2. **Blood Sugar Stabilization**: A balanced dinner helps stabilize blood sugar levels throughout the night, preventing energy crashes or disruptions in sleep.

3. **Medication Timing**: Just like with lunch, some PH medications may need to be taken with dinner. Having a substantial meal ensures that these medications are taken as prescribed and absorbed effectively.

4. **Nutrient Intake**: A nutritious dinner contributes to your overall daily intake

of essential nutrients, helping meet specific dietary requirements related to PH.

Nutritional Considerations for Heart-Healthy Dinners

Before we explore dinner ideas, let's review the key nutritional elements that should be included in a heart-healthy dinner for PH patients:

1. **Lean Protein**: Incorporate a source of lean protein to support muscle maintenance and overall strength. Options include skinless

poultry, fish, lean beef, tofu, or legumes.

2. **Complex Carbohydrates**: Whole grains like brown rice, quinoa, or whole wheat pasta provide sustained energy and are rich in fiber, which aids in digestion.

3. **Healthy Fats**: Include sources of healthy fats like avocados, nuts, or olive oil to support heart health and add flavor and richness to your dinner.

4. **Fruits and Vegetables**: Fresh or cooked vegetables and fruits are rich in vitamins, minerals, and

antioxidants, adding color and vibrancy to your dinner while supporting overall health.

5. **Low-Sodium Choices**: PH patients should remain mindful of sodium intake to manage fluid retention. Opt for low-sodium ingredients and seasonings.

PH-Friendly Dinner Ideas

Now, let's explore some PH-friendly dinner ideas that are both heart-healthy and satisfying:

1. Baked Salmon with Quinoa and Steamed Broccoli

Ingredients:

- 6 oz salmon fillet
- 1/2 cup cooked quinoa
- 1 cup steamed broccoli florets
- 1/2 lemon (sliced)
- Olive oil
- Salt and pepper to taste

Instructions:

- Preheat your oven to 375°F (190°C).
- Place the salmon fillet on a baking sheet, drizzle with olive oil, and season with salt, pepper, and lemon slices.

- Bake for 15-20 minutes until the salmon flakes easily with a fork.
- Serve with cooked quinoa and steamed broccoli.

2. Veggie Stir-Fry with Tofu

Ingredients:

- 1 cup cubed firm tofu
- 2 cups mixed stir-fry vegetables (e.g., bell peppers, broccoli, snap peas)
- 1 tablespoon low-sodium soy sauce
- 1 teaspoon sesame oil
- 1 clove garlic (minced)
- 1/2 cup cooked brown rice

Instructions:

- Heat sesame oil in a pan and add minced garlic.
- Add cubed tofu and stir-fry until lightly browned.
- Add mixed vegetables and stir-fry for an additional 5-7 minutes.
- Drizzle with low-sodium soy sauce and serve over cooked brown rice.

3. Grilled Chicken with Quinoa Salad

Ingredients:

- 6 oz grilled chicken breast
- 1 cup cooked quinoa

- 1/2 cup diced cucumbers
- 1/2 cup diced tomatoes
- 1/4 cup diced red onion
- 2 tablespoons chopped fresh parsley
- Lemon vinaigrette dressing (low-sodium)

Instructions:

- In a large bowl, combine cooked quinoa, diced cucumbers, tomatoes, red onion, and chopped parsley.
- Drizzle with lemon vinaigrette dressing and toss to coat.
- Serve with grilled chicken on top.

4. Lentil and Vegetable Stew

Ingredients:

- 1 cup cooked lentils
- 2 cups diced mixed vegetables (e.g., carrots, celery, bell peppers)
- 1 can (14 oz) low-sodium diced tomatoes
- 4 cups low-sodium vegetable broth
- 1 teaspoon olive oil
- 1 bay leaf
- Salt and pepper to taste

Instructions:

- In a large pot, heat olive oil and sauté diced vegetables until softened.
- Add cooked lentils, diced tomatoes, vegetable broth, bay leaf, salt, and pepper.
- Simmer for 20-25 minutes until vegetables are tender.

5. Quinoa and Black Bean Stuffed Bell Peppers

Ingredients:

- 2 bell peppers (any color)
- 1 cup cooked quinoa
- 1/2 cup canned black beans (rinsed and drained)
- 1/2 cup diced tomatoes

- 1/4 cup diced red onion
- 1/4 cup chopped fresh cilantro
- 1/2 teaspoon ground cumin
- Salt and pepper to taste

Instructions:

- Preheat your oven to 375°F (190°C).
- Cut the tops off the bell peppers and remove the seeds.
- In a bowl, combine cooked quinoa, black beans, diced tomatoes, red onion, cilantro, ground cumin, salt, and pepper.

- Stuff the bell peppers with the quinoa mixture and place them in a baking dish.
- Bake for 25-30 minutes until the bell peppers are tender.

These dinner ideas are designed to be both heart-healthy and PH-friendly, providing a balanced mix of nutrients and flavors while keeping sodium in check. By incorporating these meals into your dinner routine, you can support your pulmonary hypertension management while enjoying delicious, nourishing dinners.

In conclusion, Chapter 5 underscores the importance of crafting heart-healthy dinners in the context of pulmonary hypertension management. These dinner ideas offer a diverse array of flavors and ingredients, ensuring that your evening meal is both nutritious and enjoyable. As always, consult with your healthcare team for personalized dietary guidance and adjustments based on your specific needs and preferences.

CHAPTER 6

Snacks and Appetizers for PH Patients

In Chapter 6, we venture into the realm of snacks and appetizers, often overlooked components of daily nutrition. For individuals managing pulmonary hypertension (PH), choosing the right snacks and appetizers is crucial to maintain energy levels, manage hunger between meals, and support overall well-being. This chapter explores why these mini-meals are essential, delves into nutritional considerations, and provides a variety of PH-friendly snack and appetizer ideas.

The Significance of PH-Friendly Snacks and Appetizers

Snacks and appetizers serve vital roles in the daily life of someone with pulmonary hypertension:

1. **Energy Boost**: Snacks provide a quick energy boost, which is particularly important for PH patients who often experience fatigue.

2. **Hunger Management**: They help manage hunger between meals, preventing overeating at main meal times and maintaining stable blood sugar levels.

3. **Medication Compatibility**: Snack times can coincide with medication schedules, ensuring that PH medications are taken as prescribed and effectively absorbed.

4. **Nutrient Intake**: PH-friendly snacks and appetizers contribute to overall nutrient intake,

supporting specific dietary requirements related to managing the condition.

Nutritional Considerations for PH-Friendly Snacks and Appetizers

Before we delve into snack and appetizer ideas, it's essential to understand the nutritional requirements for PH patients and incorporate them into these mini-meals:

1. **Protein**: Include a source of protein in your snacks and appetizers to support muscle maintenance and overall

strength. Options include Greek yogurt, lean turkey, hummus, or edamame.

2. **Complex Carbohydrates**: Whole grains like whole wheat crackers, brown rice cakes, or whole grain bread can provide sustained energy and are rich in fiber, which aids in digestion.

3. **Healthy Fats**: Incorporate sources of healthy fats like avocado, nuts, or olive oil to support heart health and add flavor and richness to your snacks.

4. **Fruits and Vegetables**: Fresh fruits and vegetables

are excellent choices for snacks and appetizers. They are rich in vitamins, minerals, and antioxidants, adding color and vibrancy to your mini-meals while supporting overall health.

5. **Low-Sodium Options**: As with main meals, PH patients should remain mindful of sodium intake to manage fluid retention. Opt for low-sodium ingredients and seasonings.

Now, let's explore some PH-friendly snack and appetizer ideas:

1. Greek Yogurt Parfait

Ingredients:

- 1/2 cup Greek yogurt (low-fat or non-fat)
- 1/2 cup mixed berries (e.g., blueberries, raspberries)
- 1 tablespoon chopped almonds
- 1 teaspoon honey (optional)

Instructions:

- Layer Greek yogurt, mixed berries, and chopped almonds in a glass.
- Drizzle with honey for extra sweetness if desired.

2. Hummus and Veggie Sticks

Ingredients:

- 2 tablespoons hummus (low-sodium)
- Carrot sticks, cucumber slices, and bell pepper strips

Instructions:

- Dip the veggie sticks into hummus for a satisfying and crunchy snack.

3. Avocado Toast

Ingredients:

- 1 slice whole grain bread (low-sodium)
- 1/4 ripe avocado

- Sliced tomato
- Sprinkle of black pepper

Instructions:

- Toast the whole grain bread.
- Mash the ripe avocado and spread it on the toast.
- Top with sliced tomato and a sprinkle of black pepper.

4. Cottage Cheese with Pineapple

Ingredients:

- 1/2 cup low-fat cottage cheese
- 1/2 cup diced pineapple (fresh or canned in juice)

Instructions:

- Combine cottage cheese and diced pineapple for a protein-packed and fruity snack.

5. Edamame Snack

Ingredients:

- 1 cup edamame (steamed and lightly salted)
- A squeeze of fresh lemon juice

Instructions:

- Steam edamame and lightly salt them.

- Squeeze fresh lemon juice over the edamame for a zesty touch.

6. Whole Wheat Pita and Tzatziki

Ingredients:

- 1 whole wheat pita (low-sodium)
- 2 tablespoons tzatziki sauce
- Sliced cucumber and cherry tomatoes

Instructions:

- Cut the whole wheat pita into triangles.

- Serve with tzatziki sauce for dipping, along with sliced cucumber and cherry tomatoes.

These snack and appetizer ideas not only satisfy your taste buds but also align with the nutritional needs of PH patients. They offer a mix of protein, complex carbohydrates, healthy fats, and plenty of fruits and vegetables, all while keeping sodium intake in check. Incorporating these mini-meals into your daily routine can help you manage hunger, maintain energy levels, and support your overall well-being.

In conclusion, Chapter 6 underscores the importance of choosing PH-friendly snacks and appetizers to maintain a balanced diet and manage symptoms effectively. By incorporating these ideas into your daily routine, you can ensure that your mini-meals are both satisfying and nourishing. Remember to consult with your healthcare team for personalized dietary guidance tailored to your specific needs and preferences.

CHAPTER 7

PH-Safe Desserts and Sweets

In Chapter 7, we venture into the world of desserts and sweets, which can be a challenging territory for individuals managing pulmonary hypertension (PH). We'll explore why it's important to find PH-safe alternatives for indulging in something sweet, delve into nutritional considerations, and provide a variety of delicious PH-friendly dessert and sweet treat ideas.

The Role of PH-Safe Desserts and Sweets

Desserts and sweets play a significant role in our lives, offering comfort and satisfaction. For individuals managing pulmonary hypertension, it's important to strike a balance between indulging in these treats and adhering to a PH-friendly diet. Here's why:

1. **Mental Well-being**: Desserts and sweets can provide comfort and joy, which are important for mental well-being, especially

for those dealing with a chronic condition like PH.

2. **Occasional Treats**: Allowing for occasional indulgences can make adhering to a strict dietary regimen more sustainable and enjoyable.

3. **Special Occasions**: Desserts are often part of celebrations and social gatherings. Having PH-safe dessert options allows you to participate fully in these occasions.

4. **Portion Control**: Preparing PH-safe desserts at home gives you control

over portion sizes and ingredient choices, making it easier to manage sodium and other dietary concerns.

Nutritional Considerations for PH-Safe Desserts and Sweets

While it's important to enjoy desserts and sweets in moderation, there are ways to make them more PH-friendly by considering specific nutritional elements:

1. **Sodium Awareness**: PH patients should remain mindful of sodium intake,

even in desserts. Opt for low-sodium or sodium-free alternatives when possible.

2. **Sugars**: Keep an eye on added sugars, as excessive sugar intake can have negative health effects. Look for recipes that use natural sweeteners or sugar substitutes.

3. **Fiber and Whole Grains**: Incorporate whole grains and fiber-rich ingredients like oats, whole wheat flour, and fruits to add nutrients and promote digestive health.

4. **Portion Control**: Practice portion control when enjoying desserts to avoid overindulgence.

Now, let's explore some PH-friendly dessert and sweet treat ideas:

1. Fresh Fruit Salad with Honey-Lime Drizzle

Ingredients:

- Assorted fresh fruits (e.g., berries, melon, kiwi)
- 1-2 tablespoons honey (or a sugar substitute)
- Juice of 1 lime

Instructions:

- Prepare a variety of fresh fruits and arrange them in a bowl.
- In a small bowl, whisk together honey (or sugar substitute) and lime juice.
- Drizzle the honey-lime mixture over the fruit salad and gently toss to coat.

2. Baked Apples with Cinnamon

Ingredients:

- 2 apples (cored)
- 1 teaspoon cinnamon

- 1 tablespoon chopped nuts (e.g., almonds, walnuts)
- 1 teaspoon honey (or a sugar substitute)

Instructions:

- Preheat your oven to 350°F (175°C).
- Place the cored apples on a baking sheet.
- Sprinkle cinnamon over the apples and bake for 20-25 minutes until tender.
- Top with chopped nuts and a drizzle of honey (or sugar substitute) before serving.

3. Greek Yogurt and Berry Parfait

Ingredients:

- 1/2 cup Greek yogurt (low-fat or non-fat)
- 1/2 cup mixed berries (e.g., strawberries, blueberries)
- 1 tablespoon chopped almonds
- 1 teaspoon honey (optional)

Instructions:

- In a glass, layer Greek yogurt, mixed berries, and chopped almonds.
- Drizzle with honey for extra sweetness if desired.

4. Oatmeal Chocolate Chip Cookies

Ingredients:

- 1 cup rolled oats
- 1/2 cup whole wheat flour
- 1/2 cup dark chocolate chips (low-sodium)
- 1/4 cup chopped nuts (e.g., pecans, almonds)
- 1/4 cup unsweetened applesauce
- 1/4 cup honey (or a sugar substitute)
- 1/4 cup olive oil
- 1/2 teaspoon baking soda
- 1/2 teaspoon vanilla extract
- A pinch of salt

Instructions:

- Preheat your oven to 350°F (175°C) and line a baking sheet with parchment paper.
- In a bowl, combine rolled oats, whole wheat flour, dark chocolate chips, chopped nuts, baking soda, and a pinch of salt.
- In a separate bowl, whisk together unsweetened applesauce, honey (or sugar substitute), olive oil, and vanilla extract.
- Pour the wet ingredients into the dry ingredients and mix until combined.

- Drop spoonfuls of the cookie dough onto the prepared baking sheet.
- Bake for 10-12 minutes or until the edges are golden brown.

5. Banana Ice Cream

Ingredients:

- 2 ripe bananas
- 1/4 cup unsweetened almond milk (or your choice of milk)
- 1 teaspoon vanilla extract
- Optional toppings: chopped nuts, dark chocolate chips,

or a drizzle of honey (or a sugar substitute)

Instructions:

- Slice ripe bananas and freeze them until solid.
- Place the frozen banana slices, almond milk, and vanilla extract in a blender or food processor.
- Blend until smooth and creamy.
- Serve immediately with your choice of toppings.

These dessert and sweet treat ideas offer a delightful balance between indulgence and health consciousness. They incorporate fresh fruits, whole grains, and natural sweeteners, making them suitable for PH patients while satisfying your sweet cravings.

In conclusion, Chapter 7 highlights the importance of finding PH-friendly alternatives for desserts and sweet treats. By incorporating these ideas into your dietary routine, you can enjoy occasional indulgences while supporting your overall health and well-being. As always, consult with your healthcare team for personalized dietary guidance and adjustments based on your specific needs and preferences.

CHAPTER 8

PH-Safe Beverages

In Chapter 8, we dive into the world of beverages, often an overlooked aspect of dietary management for individuals dealing with pulmonary hypertension (PH). We'll explore the significance of choosing the right beverages, delve into the nutritional considerations, and provide a variety of PH-friendly beverage options that can help you stay hydrated and support your overall well-being.

The Importance of PH-Safe Beverages

Beverages are an integral part of daily life, providing hydration and flavor. For PH patients, it's essential to consider beverage choices for several reasons:

1. **Hydration**: Proper hydration is crucial for everyone, but especially for PH patients, as dehydration can exacerbate symptoms like fatigue and dizziness.

2. **Medication Compatibility**: Some PH medications may require you to drink fluids with them.

Choosing the right beverages ensures you can take your medications as prescribed.

3. **Sodium Control**: Managing sodium intake is vital for PH patients to prevent fluid retention. Careful selection of low-sodium beverages is essential.

4. **Nutrient Support**: Beverages can contribute to your overall nutrient intake. Opting for PH-safe choices helps you meet your dietary requirements while managing your condition.

Nutritional Considerations for PH-Safe Beverages

When it comes to selecting PH-safe beverages, there are key nutritional elements to consider:

1. **Sodium Content**: Check the sodium content on beverage labels and opt for low-sodium or sodium-free options when possible.

2. **Sugars**: Be mindful of added sugars in beverages, as excessive sugar intake can have negative health effects. Choose beverages with little or no added sugars.

3. **Hydration**: Hydrating beverages like water and herbal teas should be your primary choices for maintaining proper hydration.

4. **Caffeine**: While some caffeine is generally safe, excessive caffeine intake can lead to increased heart rate and blood pressure. Monitor your caffeine intake, and if in doubt, consult your healthcare team.

5. **Alcohol**: Moderate alcohol consumption may be acceptable for some PH patients, but it's essential to

consult with your healthcare provider to determine if it's safe for you.

Now, let's explore some PH-friendly beverage options:

1. Water

Water is the most crucial beverage for hydration, and it should be the primary choice for PH patients. Staying adequately hydrated helps manage symptoms like fatigue and dizziness.

2. Herbal Teas

Herbal teas, such as chamomile, peppermint, or ginger tea, are caffeine-free options that can be soothing and hydrating. Be sure to check for any herbal teas that may interact with your medications and consult your healthcare team if you have concerns.

3. Coconut Water

Coconut water is a natural source of electrolytes and can be a hydrating choice. Look for unsweetened varieties with no added sodium.

4. Infused Water

Enhance the flavor of your water by adding slices of fruits, vegetables, or herbs. Try combinations like cucumber and mint, lemon and ginger, or strawberry and basil.

5. Low-Sodium Vegetable Juice

If you enjoy the taste of vegetable juice, look for low-sodium varieties. These can provide vitamins and minerals without excessive sodium intake.

6. Smoothies

Homemade smoothies can be a nutritious and enjoyable way to hydrate. Use ingredients like frozen fruits, Greek yogurt (low-fat or non-fat), and a splash of almond milk (unsweetened) for a refreshing treat.

7. Lemon Water

A squeeze of fresh lemon juice in water can add a burst of flavor without added sugars. Lemon water can also promote digestion and provide a source of vitamin C.

8. Decaffeinated Coffee or Tea

If you enjoy coffee or tea, opt for decaffeinated versions to minimize caffeine intake. Also, consider herbal teas or caffeine-free blends.

9. Fruit-Infused Sparkling Water

For a fizzy treat, choose unsweetened, fruit-infused sparkling water. These beverages come in various flavors without added sugars.

10. Low-Alcohol or Alcohol-Free Beer and Wine (if approved by your healthcare team)

In some cases, PH patients may be able to enjoy low-alcohol or alcohol-free versions of beer and wine. Always consult your healthcare provider before consuming alcohol to ensure it's safe for your condition.

11. Homemade Electrolyte Drink

If you're looking to replenish electrolytes after exercise or on hot days, consider making a homemade electrolyte drink using ingredients like water, a pinch of salt, a squeeze of lemon or lime juice, and a touch of honey (or a sugar substitute).

These beverage options offer a range of choices for PH patients, ensuring proper hydration and enjoyment without compromising dietary restrictions. Whether you prefer simple water, herbal infusions, or occasional treats like smoothies, you can find suitable options that align with your health needs.

In conclusion, Chapter 8 emphasizes the importance of choosing PH-safe beverages to support hydration and overall well-being. By incorporating these beverage choices into your daily routine, you can stay properly hydrated while managing your condition. Always consult with your healthcare team for personalized guidance on your dietary choices, including beverages, based on your specific needs and preferences.

CHAPTER 9

Dining Out with PH

In Chapter 9, we tackle the challenges and opportunities of dining out for individuals managing pulmonary hypertension (PH). Eating out can be a source of enjoyment and social connection, but it also requires careful consideration to maintain a PH-friendly diet. This chapter explores why dining out matters, offers strategies for navigating restaurant menus, and provides tips for a successful dining experience while managing your condition.

The Importance of Dining Out with PH

Dining out is more than just a meal; it's a social and cultural experience. For PH patients, it's essential for several reasons:

1. **Social Interaction**: Dining out allows you to connect with friends and family, fostering social well-being, which is vital for mental health.

2. **Variety and Enjoyment**: It provides variety and

enjoyment in your diet, making it easier to stick to your PH-friendly eating plan in the long run.

3. **Special Occasions**: Celebratory events often involve dining out. Learning how to navigate restaurant menus ensures you can participate fully in these occasions.

4. **Convenience**: Sometimes, dining out is the most convenient option. Knowing how to make informed choices at restaurants can help you maintain your dietary restrictions.

Strategies for Dining Out with PH

Navigating restaurant menus as a PH patient can be challenging, but it's entirely possible with the right strategies:

1. **Research the Restaurant**: Before choosing a restaurant, review their menu online if available. Look for dishes that align with your dietary needs, such as those with lean protein, low sodium, and whole grains.

2. **Call Ahead**: Don't hesitate to call the restaurant in

advance. Ask if they can accommodate specific dietary requests or if they have any low-sodium options available.

3. **Ask Questions**: When you arrive at the restaurant, don't be shy about asking questions. Inquire about how dishes are prepared, whether they can be customized, and if sodium can be reduced.

4. **Be Mindful of Sodium**: Sodium can be hidden in sauces, dressings, and seasonings. Request sauces and dressings on the side,

and ask for sodium-free seasonings or lemon wedges as flavor enhancers.

5. **Portion Control**: Restaurant portions are often larger than what you need. Consider sharing a dish or taking leftovers home to avoid overeating.

6. **Customize Your Order**: Many restaurants are willing to customize dishes. For example, you can request grilled instead of fried, or substitute sides like French fries with steamed vegetables.

7. **Avoid Buffets**: Buffet-style dining can be challenging to navigate due to limited control over ingredients and portion sizes. It's often best to choose restaurants with a la carte menus.

Tips for Specific Types of Cuisine

Different types of cuisine may present unique challenges and opportunities for PH patients:

- **Italian**: Opt for pasta dishes with tomato-based sauces (marinara), and ask for whole wheat pasta when available. Avoid creamy sauces and dishes high in cheese.

- **Asian**: Choose steamed or stir-fried dishes with lean protein, such as chicken, tofu, or seafood. Be cautious of soy sauce, which is high in sodium, and request low-sodium alternatives.

- **Mexican**: Opt for dishes like grilled chicken fajitas or soft tacos with lean protein and plenty of vegetables. Ask for salsa and guacamole on the side to control portions.

- **American**: Look for grilled options on the menu, such as grilled chicken or fish, and ask for vegetables or a salad as a side. Avoid fried foods and dishes with heavy gravies.

Strategies for Coping with Dietary Restrictions

Dining out with PH may sometimes require creative strategies:

- **Share Your Needs**: Inform your dining companions about your dietary restrictions so they can choose a restaurant that accommodates your needs.

- **BYO**: In some cases, you can bring your own low-sodium condiments or seasonings to enhance the flavor of your meal.

- **Plan Ahead**: If you know you'll be dining out, adjust your other meals for the day to accommodate the restaurant meal.

Mindful Eating Practices

Beyond choosing the right foods, practicing mindful eating can enhance your dining-out experience:

- **Savor Your Food**: Take your time to enjoy each bite, focusing on the flavors and textures. This can help you feel more satisfied with smaller portions.

- **Listen to Your Body**: Pay attention to your body's hunger and fullness cues. Stop eating when you're satisfied, not overly full.

- **Stay Hydrated**: Drink water throughout your meal to aid digestion and help you recognize feelings of fullness.

- **Limit Distractions**: Put away your phone or other

distractions to fully engage with your meal and the people you're dining with.

Managing Desserts and Beverages

When it comes to dessert and beverages while dining out:

- **Desserts**: Choose desserts wisely, opting for fruit-based options, sorbet, or sharing a dessert with others to control portion sizes.

- **Beverages**: Be mindful of beverage choices, selecting water, herbal tea, or unsweetened options to avoid excessive sugar and caffeine.

Plan for Special Occasions

For special occasions, you can plan ahead to make dining out enjoyable and PH-friendly:

- **Review the Menu in Advance**: Know what you'll order to avoid making impulsive choices.
- **Communicate Your Needs**: Inform the server about your dietary restrictions and ask for modifications as needed.

- **Control Portions**: Consider sharing an appetizer or dessert to balance your meal.
- **Enjoy the Company**: Focus on the social aspect of dining out rather than just the food. Engage in meaningful conversations with your companions.

In conclusion, Chapter 9 emphasizes the importance of dining out as a PH patient and provides practical strategies for making the experience enjoyable while maintaining dietary restrictions. By planning ahead, asking questions, and practicing mindful eating, you can savor delicious meals and participate fully in social occasions without compromising your health. Always consult with your healthcare team for personalized dietary guidance based on your specific needs and preferences.

CHAPTER 10

PH-Friendly Meal Planning and Conclusion

In Chapter 10, we'll explore the crucial aspects of meal planning and conclude our journey through the world of pulmonary hypertension (PH) dietary management. Meal planning is the cornerstone of maintaining a PH-friendly diet consistently, and it helps individuals with PH stay on track with their dietary restrictions while enjoying a variety of nourishing foods. This final chapter will provide you with practical guidance on meal planning and offer a concluding perspective on your PH journey.

The Significance of PH-Friendly Meal Planning

Meal planning is a structured approach to selecting, preparing, and enjoying meals that align with your dietary requirements. For PH patients, meal planning holds several key benefits:

1. **Consistency**: Meal planning ensures that you consistently follow your PH-

friendly diet, reducing the risk of accidental deviations.

2. **Variety**: Planning your meals allows you to incorporate a diverse range of foods, preventing dietary monotony.

3. **Nutrient Balance**: You can carefully balance your nutrient intake, ensuring that you meet your specific dietary needs while managing your condition.

4. **Portion Control**: Meal planning helps you control portion sizes, which is crucial for avoiding

overeating and managing sodium intake.

5. **Time and Stress Management**: Preparing a meal plan reduces the stress of deciding what to eat daily and saves time on grocery shopping and meal preparation.

Creating a PH-Friendly Meal Plan

Creating a meal plan tailored to your PH needs involves several steps:

1. Consult Your Healthcare Team: Before crafting your meal

plan, consult with your healthcare provider and a registered dietitian. They can provide personalized guidance based on your specific condition and dietary restrictions.

2. Identify Dietary Restrictions: Clearly understand your dietary restrictions, including sodium, fluid intake, and other specific recommendations provided by your healthcare team.

3. Set Meal Frequencies: Determine how many meals and snacks you'll have each day. Regular, balanced meals and snacks can help stabilize blood sugar levels and maintain energy.

4. Choose PH-Friendly Foods: Select foods that align with your dietary restrictions and are PH-friendly. These may include lean proteins, whole grains, fruits, vegetables, and low-sodium options.

5. Balance Nutrients: Ensure that each meal contains a balance of nutrients, including protein, complex carbohydrates, healthy fats, and fiber. This balance supports overall health and symptom management.

6. Monitor Portions: Be mindful of portion sizes, especially for foods high in sodium. Using measuring cups and utensils can help with portion control.

7. Plan for Special Occasions: When dining out or attending special events, plan your meals and snacks accordingly to accommodate these occasions without compromising your dietary restrictions.

8. Create a Shopping List: Based on your meal plan, compile a shopping list of the ingredients you'll need. This list streamlines grocery shopping and minimizes impulse purchases.

9. Prepare Ahead: Consider batch cooking or preparing components of meals in advance to save time during the week. Having prepped ingredients readily available makes sticking to your meal plan easier.

10. Be Flexible: While meal planning provides structure, it's essential to remain flexible. Life can be unpredictable, so be open to adjustments when needed.

Sample PH-Friendly Meal Plan

Here's a sample PH-friendly meal plan for a day:

Breakfast:

- Scrambled eggs with diced tomatoes and spinach
- Whole wheat toast (low-sodium)
- Fresh fruit salad (e.g., berries, melon)

Mid-Morning Snack:

- Greek yogurt (low-fat or non-fat)
- A sprinkle of chopped nuts and honey (or a sugar substitute)

Lunch:

- Grilled chicken breast salad with mixed greens, cherry tomatoes, cucumber, and a vinaigrette dressing (low-sodium)
- Quinoa or brown rice on the side

Afternoon Snack:

- Sliced bell peppers and cucumber with hummus (low-sodium)

Dinner:

- Baked salmon with lemon and dill
- Steamed broccoli and carrots

- Mashed sweet potatoes (without added salt)

Evening Snack (if needed):

- A small portion of fruit or a handful of unsalted nuts

CONCLUSION

and Reflecting on Your PH Journey

As we conclude our exploration of PH-friendly meal planning, it's essential to reflect on your journey managing pulmonary hypertension. Living with a chronic condition like PH requires dedication and self-care, and your dietary choices play a significant role in your overall well-being.

Here are some key takeaways to remember:

1. Consult Your Healthcare Team: Your healthcare provider, pulmonologist, and registered dietitian are invaluable resources for managing PH. Regular check-ups and open communication with your healthcare team are essential.

2. Knowledge Empowers: Understanding your condition and its dietary implications empowers you to make informed choices. Educate yourself about PH and ask questions when needed.

3. Support Matters: Building a support network of friends and family who understand your condition and dietary restrictions can provide emotional and practical assistance on your journey.

4. Self-Care is Vital: Managing PH requires self-care in various forms, including regular exercise (as advised by your healthcare team), stress management, and adhering to your dietary plan.

5. Embrace Variety: While PH imposes dietary restrictions, there's still room for variety and enjoyment in your meals. Explore different recipes, cuisines, and cooking methods to keep your meals interesting.

6. Be Mindful of Balance: Balancing your dietary needs with enjoyment is a lifelong endeavor. It's okay to occasionally indulge in moderation but remember the importance of consistency.

7. Stay Informed: Medical research and treatments for PH continue to evolve. Stay informed about the latest developments in PH management and discuss them with your healthcare team.

8. Celebrate Your Achievements: Managing a chronic condition like PH can be challenging, but celebrate your achievements, no matter how small. Each day you adhere to your dietary plan is a victory.

In conclusion, creating and maintaining a PH-friendly meal plan is a vital aspect of managing your condition. It empowers you to make dietary choices that support your health and well-being while still enjoying a variety of delicious foods. Remember that your journey with PH is unique, and by working closely with your healthcare team and adopting a mindful approach to nutrition, you can lead a fulfilling life while managing your condition.